FROM MANAGING TO CONQUERING ERECTILE DYSFUNCTION

Expert Guide To Understanding the Causes, Recognizing Symptoms, and Embracing Effective Treatments for a Vibrant and Healthy Life

DR. DASHIELL DANIEL

Disclaimer

This book, is intended to provide information and guidance on the subject matter and is not a substitute for professional medical advice, diagnosis, or treatment.

The author, is not a medical professional, and the content presented here is based on research, general knowledge, and expert guidance available at the time of writing.

The information in this book is provided with the understanding that the author and the publisher are not engaged in rendering medical, legal, or other professional services.

Any reliance on the information contained in this book is at the reader's own risk.

While every effort has been made to ensure the accuracy and completeness of the information presented, medical knowledge is constantly evolving, and new research may supersede the content in this book. The author and the publisher make no representations or warranties of any kind, express or implied, about the completeness, accuracy, reliability, suitability, or availability concerning the information, products, services, or related graphics contained in this book.

This book may contain references or mentions of individuals, products, websites, organizations, or other names for informational purposes only.

The author does not own or endorse any such entities mentioned in the book. Any resemblance to actual persons, living or dead, or actual events is purely coincidental.

Readers are encouraged to consult with qualified healthcare professionals for medical advice, diagnosis, and treatment tailored to their specific circumstances.

The author and the publisher disclaim any liability for any loss or risk, personal or otherwise, arising directly or indirectly from the use of the information presented in this book.

By reading this book, the reader acknowledges and agrees to the terms of this disclaimer.

The book "Erectile Dysfunction" tackles a serious and widespread health problem that has a big influence on people's relationships and general well-being. Its thorough examination of the topic gives readers a deep understanding of erectile dysfunction (ED) and all of its facets, which is why it is so important. The first section acts as a starting point by highlighting the importance of addressing and recognizing ED for relational dynamics as well as personal health.

In Chapter 1, the basics of ED are covered, including its definition, causes, and dispelling common myths. Understanding the fundamentals of ED is essential for readers to be able to differentiate between the medical, psychological, and lifestyle elements that contribute to the condition's expression.

Subsequently, Chapter 2 describes the telltale signs and symptoms of eating disorders (ED), classifying them into several forms and emphasizing the significant effects they have on relationships and mental health. The next chapters walk readers through the steps of getting professional assistance, stressing the need of working together to diagnose and develop treatments.

The therapy modalities—which range from medical interventions to lifestyle changes, psychological methods, and natural remedies—are thoroughly examined in Chapters 4 through 7. The inclusion of thorough analyses of drugs, surgical procedures, and holistic approaches gives readers a wide range of information to help them make decisions about their health.

In Chapter 8, the need of long-term lifestyle modifications for general health is emphasized. Topics covered include quitting smoking, consuming alcohol in moderation, and managing weight. In order to manage the complexities of relationships impacted by ED, Chapter 9 places a strong emphasis on open communication, intimacy that goes beyond sex, and the possible advantages of relationship counseling.

Chapter 10, which closes the book, provides insight into how ED treatments will develop moving forward by highlighting new treatments and continuing research. This forward-looking viewpoint guarantees that readers are aware of both prospective developments in the subject and present options.

"Erectile Dysfunction" is essentially a thorough manual that delves deeper beyond the surface, giving readers the skills they need to comprehend, control, and conquer ED. Its well-structured and scholarly tone encourage a scholarly approach to a subject having broad significance for the well-being of individuals and relationships.

Overview

One of the most common medical conditions impacting a large number of men globally is erectile dysfunction (ED).

This thorough manual seeks to explore many facets of overcoming erectile dysfunction, offering insightful knowledge on the comprehension and treatment of this illness. People can develop a more nuanced understanding of ED's causes, consequences, and the significance of treating it for both physical and psychological well-being by investigating the many facets of the disorder.

Concerning This Book

This manual provides an assortment of research-backed data, medical knowledge, and useful tactics to assist people in their quest to overcome erectile dysfunction. It provides a comprehensive and knowledgeable approach by drawing on a wide range of sources, such as medical literature, professional viewpoints, and firsthand experiences. The book is designed to meet the needs of readers who want a thorough understanding of ED, its causes, and the variety of strategies that can be used to effectively manage and treat this illness. It is a thorough guide for anybody attempting to understand the nuances of erectile dysfunction.

Knowledge Of Erectile Dysfunction

The inability to consistently get or sustain an erection strong enough for sexual activity is known as erectile dysfunction, a complex medical problem. It is caused by a confluence of behavioral, psychological, and physiological variables. From a physiological standpoint, ED may be associated with vascular problems, hormone abnormalities, or neurological conditions that impact the complex mechanisms underlying penile function. Relationship dynamics, stress, anxiety, and depression are psychological factors that can influence how ED appears and persists. The complex interactions between these elements will be thoroughly examined in this portion of the guide, providing insight into the psychological and physiological causes of erectile dysfunction.

Treating Erectile Dysfunction Is Critical

Erectile dysfunction affects sexual performance immediately, but it also has wider effects on general health and wellbeing.

Relationship problems, low self-esteem, and emotional anguish are common among those with ED. Furthermore, ED may signal the presence of underlying medical disorders such diabetes, cardiovascular disease, or hormone imbalances. Treating ED is a comprehensive effort that aims to improve mental health, promote good relationships, and stop the advancement of related medical issues in addition to just restoring sexual function. This section will elaborate on the significance of identifying erectile dysfunction and actively pursuing treatments, stressing the condition's function as a gauge for more serious health issues.

this article aims to give readers a thorough grasp of erectile dysfunction by examining its complex nature and highlighting the importance of treating this illness. People can learn more about aspects of health and well-being that go beyond the bedroom by exploring the physiological and psychological complexities of ED. By providing information, techniques, and a feeling of agency, this site seeks to enable people to overcome erectile dysfunction and recover a happy, healthy life.

CHAPTER ONE
THE ESSENTIALS OF ERECTILE DYSFUNCTION

Definition and Synopsis: The persistent inability to get or sustain an erection strong enough for sexual activity is the hallmark of erectile dysfunction (ED), a common medical disease.

The impacted people's and their partners' quality of life is greatly impacted. The disorder is caused by a complex interaction of lifestyle, psychological, and physical variables rather than being a direct result of aging.

A person with ED may experience varying degrees of symptoms, from infrequent trouble getting an erection to total incapacity to participate in sexual activities. It is essential to comprehend the complex nature of ED in order to create preventative and treatment plans that work.

Erectile Dysfunction Causes

Physical variables: There are several physical variables that play a major role in the development of ED. Atherosclerosis and hypertension are two vascular conditions that can reduce blood flow to the penile area, making it more difficult to get and keep an erection.

Multiple sclerosis and Parkinson's disease are two neurological disorders that can interfere with the complex signaling pathways that are involved in the erectile response. ED may be exacerbated by hormonal abnormalities, especially low testosterone levels. A thorough medical evaluation is essential to determine and treat any underlying physical problems, as some drugs, including antidepressants and antihypertensives, have been linked to the problem.

Psychological causes: ED is frequently caused by psychological causes, and the mind-body connection is crucial to sexual function.

Stress, worry, and sadness can impair a person's ability to get an erection by upsetting the delicate neurotransmitter balance. Fear of sexual inadequacy at the core of performance anxiety can lead to a self-fulfilling prophesy, so aggravating ED. Psychological impediments that impede sexual function can also be attributed to relationship problems and a lack of emotional connection.

Understanding and treating these psychological aspects is necessary for all-encompassing ED care.

Lifestyle Factors: Sexual function and general health are significantly impacted by lifestyle decisions. There is a correlation between smoking, binge drinking, and using illegal drugs and a higher chance of developing ED. Obesity and sedentary lives lead to poor cardiovascular health, which is closely related to erectile dysfunction. In order to prevent and treat ED, leading a healthy lifestyle that includes regular exercise, a balanced diet, and giving up bad habits might be quite important.

A thorough treatment strategy that incorporates lifestyle changes can greatly enhance overall sexual health.

Common Myths: There are a number of common myths about ED that can make it difficult to properly comprehend and treat the illness. One widespread misunderstanding is that ED is a necessary component of aging.

Although the increased prevalence of underlying health issues with age can be a contributing factor, ED is not a natural outcome of aging. Another myth is that eating disorders are only physical in nature. As was previously mentioned, lifestyle and psychological factors are important in the onset and aggravation of ED. In order to promote a more accurate and nuanced knowledge of the disorder and, eventually, more successful preventative and treatment efforts, it is imperative that these myths be dispelled.

To sum up, erectile dysfunction is a complex disorder with a variety of underlying causes. Creating comprehensive plans to prevent and treat ED requires an understanding of the intricate interactions that exist between lifestyle, psychological, and physical factors. Healthcare professionals and individuals can collaborate to improve overall well-being and promote sexual health by addressing the underlying reasons and dispelling prevalent myths.

CHAPTER TWO
IDENTIFYING THE SYMPTOMS AND SIGNS

Early intervention and successful treatment of erectile dysfunction (ED) depend heavily on the ability to recognize its indications and symptoms. Having trouble getting or keeping an erection on occasion is a common early warning indication. Males may experience erections that are of lower quality or that last for less time when they are stiff. Despite their subtlety, these early warning signs are significant indications that demand attention.

A decreased libido or a lack of interest in sexual activities are two further symptoms that could point to underlying problems impacting sexual function. In order to enable prompt diagnosis and action, it is imperative that both individuals and healthcare professionals exercise caution when recognizing these early indicators.

Erectile Dysfunction Types

Developing successful treatment plans requires an awareness of the varied varieties of erectile dysfunction, which is a complex disorder with a variety of underlying reasons. Physical conditions including diabetes, cardiovascular disease, or hormonal abnormalities that prevent blood flow to the penis are the root cause of organic erectile dysfunction. Conversely, psychogenic erectile dysfunction is mainly caused by psychological factors including interpersonal problems, stress, or anxiety. Understanding these differences is essential to modifying therapy strategies to target the unique factors causing the patient's ED. A thorough knowledge of the various forms of erectile dysfunction serves as the basis for a customized and focused treatment strategy.

Synthetic Dysfunction Of The Penis

The complex process of getting and keeping an erection is interfered with by physiological variables that cause organic erectile dysfunction. An erection may be difficult to obtain due to vascular problems such as peripheral vascular disease, hypertension, and atherosclerosis that impair blood flow to the penis. Another major organic cause is diabetes, a disorder that impairs blood circulation and nerve function.

Organic erectile dysfunction can also be caused by hormonal abnormalities, namely low testosterone levels. For the purpose of making an accurate diagnosis and developing successful treatment plans that may include lifestyle changes, medication, or surgery, a thorough study of these physical aspects is essential.

Insane Prostatic Hyperfunction

The underlying cause of psychogenic erectile dysfunction is psychological interference with sexual arousal and performance. Relationship problems, stress, worry, and depression are major causes of this kind of ED. Treating psychogenic erectile dysfunction requires an understanding of the complex interactions that exist between the mind and sexual function. To address underlying emotional and relational concerns, therapeutic approaches may include couples' therapy, psychiatric counseling, or stress management strategies. A comprehensive approach to treatment is made possible by realizing the psychosocial factors at work and the intricate relationship between sexual function and mental health.

Effects On Mental Health And Relationships

In addition to having a negative impact on a person's physical health, erectile dysfunction also has a significant negative impact on relationships and mental health. The inability to have fulfilling sexual relations might cause feelings of shame, inadequacy, or frustration, all of which can exacerbate the fall in self-esteem. Relationship tension can result from partners' emotional distress and frustration. The influence on psychological well-being might encompass ailments like anxiety and sadness. Understanding these effects is essential for an all-encompassing treatment strategy for ED, which should address the psychological and social effects in addition to the physiological ones.

Open communication, couples' therapy, and psychological support can all be essential parts of a comprehensive treatment strategy that aims to restore emotional and sexual well-being.

overcoming erectile dysfunction necessitates a sophisticated comprehension of its manifestations, varieties, and wider ramifications.

Early detection of warning indicators enables prompt intervention, avoiding the condition's worsening.

Differentiating between psychogenic and biological elements helps to create focused therapy plans. Furthermore, realizing the effects on relationships and mental health highlights the necessity of a comprehensive strategy that takes into account the condition's many facets.

To effectively manage erectile dysfunction and restore overall well-being, a thorough and tailored treatment strategy that takes into account both psychological and physical components is necessary.

CHAPTER THREE
SEEKING PROFESSIONAL ASSISTANCE

Seeking expert assistance can provide comfort and practical solutions for those suffering from erectile dysfunction. Realizing how crucial medical professionals are to the management and treatment of erectile dysfunction is the first step in overcoming it. In order to guide people through a comprehensive procedure that includes an initial consultation, a thorough diagnosis, and a collaborative approach to therapy, healthcare experts are essential. People can move toward a healthier and more satisfying sexual life by realizing the importance of getting expert assistance.

The Function Of Medical Professionals

Urologists, endocrinologists, and sexual health specialists are among the medical professionals who play a crucial role in treating and curing erectile dysfunction. These specialists have the skills and information needed to evaluate, diagnose, and create efficient treatment programs. Particularly trained in the male reproductive system, urologists are ideally suited to investigate the physiological underpinnings of erectile dysfunction. Endocrinologists focus on hormone imbalances that may be a contributing factor to the ailment, offering an endocrine perspective. Specialists in sexual health offer a comprehensive approach that takes psychological and physiological aspects into account. Working together, these medical professionals give a thorough and interdisciplinary approach to treating erectile dysfunction.

First Consultation And Assessment

The foundation of the process is the initial consultation, which gives medical professionals important information about the patient's medical background, way of life, and possible causes of erectile dysfunction.

Healthcare practitioners establish a secure environment for patients to talk about their worries and experiences by communicating with them in an open and nonjudgmental manner. By establishing the groundwork for a comprehensive diagnosis, this conversation enables medical professionals to pinpoint the underlying reasons and modify treatment regimens accordingly.

Health Background

An essential part of the first visit is getting a comprehensive medical history. Medical professionals investigate the patient's past and current health issues, prescription drugs, lifestyle choices, and any psychological stressors that might affect their ability to conceive. Comprehending the medical history of the patient facilitates the identification of potential risk factors and causative aspects, hence enabling healthcare practitioners to develop a customized and efficacious treatment plan.

Physical Inspection

A physical examination is a crucial step in the diagnosis procedure. In evaluating the patient's general health, medical professionals pay particular attention to the patient's endocrine and cardiovascular systems, as well as their genital and neurological systems. Physical examinations help to detect any neurological deficits, circulatory problems, or anatomical abnormalities that may be associated with erectile dysfunction. This thorough assessment offers insightful information that helps with a more precise diagnosis and focused treatment.

Diagnostic Examinations

To learn more about the underlying reasons of erectile dysfunction, diagnostic testing may be advised in some situations.

Endocrine abnormalities and metabolic problems can be revealed by blood tests that measure blood glucose, cholesterol, and hormone levels.

To evaluate blood flow and find any structural anomalies, imaging tests like nocturnal penile tumescence testing or penile Doppler ultrasonography may also be used. By improving the accuracy of the diagnosis, these diagnostic techniques guarantee that treatment regimens target the particular causes of erectile dysfunction.

Teamwork In The Treatment Process

Treating erectile dysfunction calls for a team-based, patient-focused approach to care. Healthcare professionals collaborate closely with patients to create individualized plans that include dietary changes, psychological counseling, and, if needed, prescription medication.

Dietary adjustments, consistent exercise, and stress reduction methods are examples of lifestyle improvements that can enhance one's general well-being and sexual health.

A key component of treatment is psychological support, which recognizes the interaction of the mind and body in sexual function. When it comes to treating underlying psychological factors that contribute to erectile dysfunction, marital problems, or performance anxiety, counseling and psychotherapy can be extremely helpful. In order to give a thorough and integrated approach to care, mental health specialists and healthcare practitioners work together.

Pharmaceutical interventions, including inhibitors of phosphodiesterase type 5 (PDE5), are a commonly used treatment for erectile dysfunction. Erections are made easier by medications such as vardenafil, tadalafil, and sildenafil, which increase blood flow to the penis. Based on the patient's health situation, preferences, and medication interactions, healthcare experts carefully evaluate whether these medications are appropriate. Certain situations or preferences may call for the use of alternative therapies, such as penile injections or vacuum erection equipment.

In summary, overcoming erectile dysfunction requires initiative, and getting treatment from a specialist is a crucial first step.

Healthcare professionals use their skills to help patients through a rigorous procedure that includes an initial consultation, a detailed diagnosis, and a team-based treatment plan. People can manage the complexity of erectile dysfunction and work toward a full and satisfied sexual life by comprehending the role of healthcare providers, respecting the importance of the initial consultation and diagnosis, and embracing a collaborative treatment strategy.

CHAPTER FOUR
MEDICAL TREATMENTS

A common disorder that can have a major negative influence on a person's quality of life is erectile dysfunction (ED). Medical treatments are one of the most important ways to manage ED since they target the physiological causes that underlie this illness.

Oral drugs: Using oral drugs to treat erectile dysfunction is one of the most popular and extensively recommended treatments. Notably, phosphodiesterase type 5 (PDE5) inhibitors are a class of pharmacological medicines that includes Levitra, Cialis, and Viagra. These medications function by amplifying the effects of nitric oxide, a substance that relaxes penile muscles and increases blood flow. Differentiating between the onset and duration of action, Viagra (sildenafil), Cialis (tadalafil), and Levitra (vardenafil) have all shown efficacy in several clinical trials.

Even though these drugs are usually well taken, headache, flushing, and gastrointestinal discomfort are only a few of the possible adverse effects. To maximize the use of these drugs in the treatment of ED, it is essential to comprehend the pharmacokinetics and unique patient profiles.

Injections and suppositories: These provide an alternate therapeutic method for people who don't respond well to oral drugs or can't take them because of certain contraindications.

Vasodilators like alprostadil are injected directly into the penile tissue during intravenous injections. In order to enhance blood flow to the penis, alprostadil-containing intraurethral suppositories can also be placed into the urethra.

Despite their effectiveness, these techniques could necessitate a certain degree of patient comfort with self-administration and might result in local side effects including discomfort or priapism. Therefore, using injections and suppositories in the management of ED requires appropriate patient education and supervision.

Vacuum Erection Devices: For those looking for non-invasive alternatives to pharmaceutical therapies, vacuum erection devices (VEDs) provide a choice. In order to facilitate an erection, these devices work by producing a vacuum surrounding the penis, which draws blood into the erectile tissues. To sustain the erection, VEDs are made up of a constriction ring that is positioned at the base of the penis, a cylinder, and a pump. Even though VEDs are usually well accepted, some people may find them difficult to use, or they may cause pain or bruises. To maximize the benefits of vacuum erection devices, patient counseling and appropriate device usage instructions are essential.

Surgical Options: Surgical operations may be taken into consideration for patients who do not respond to conservative or less invasive therapy. Devices that are surgically inserted into the penis to facilitate an erection are referred to as penile implants, or penile prostheses.

Semi-rigid and inflatable penile implants are the two primary varieties. Semi-rigid implants keep a consistent firmness, whereas inflatable implants facilitate fluid movement between reservoirs for a more natural erection. Penile implant patient satisfaction rates are generally excellent, although surgery carries dangers of its own, such as infection and mechanical failure.

Another surgical approach for treating erectile dysfunction is vascular surgery, especially if arterial insufficiency is the underlying cause.

This method seeks to revascularize the arterial supply in order to increase blood flow to the penis. Vascular surgery is not as widely used as other treatments, although it might be a good choice for some patients with particular vascular problems. The patient should be adequately informed about the possible results and consequences connected with vascular surgery for ED, and the risks and advantages of such operations must be carefully weighed.

In conclusion, the variety of medical interventions available for erectile dysfunction is a reflection of both the condition's complexity and the wide range of demands of those who experience it.

Every erection method—vacuum erection devices, injections, oral drugs, and surgery—has advantages and downsides of its own.

Achieving the best possible results in the management of erectile dysfunction requires customizing the treatment plan for each patient, taking into account personal preferences and comorbidities. Furthermore, continuous research and scientific developments in the field of medicine contribute to the improvement and diversification of treatment options, providing hope for a better quality of life for those impacted by this prevalent and significant illness.

CHAPTER FIVE
CHANGES IN LIFESTYLE

A multimodal strategy is typically necessary for the efficient management of erectile dysfunction (ED), with lifestyle adjustments being a critical component. Dietary changes are a crucial component. For general health, a well-balanced, nutrient-rich diet is essential, and certain foods have been linked to promoting sexual health. Fruits, vegetables, whole grains, and lean proteins are among the foods that can have a good effect on vascular health, which is essential for erectile performance. Berries and leafy greens are two examples of foods high in antioxidants that help vasodilate and may lessen oxidative stress, which is linked to ED. On the other hand, one cannot ignore the impact of eating habits that are harmful to one's sexual health. Obesity and vascular dysfunction are risk factors for eating disorders that have been related to overindulgence in processed foods, sweets, and saturated fats. Therefore, implementing a nutritionally balanced diet becomes essential to the overall management of ED.

In addition to food modifications, engaging in regular physical activity is another essential lifestyle change. Exercise directly contributes to improved vascular health in addition to helping with weight management. Exercises that are specifically aerobic in nature, in particular, improve blood circulation, which in turn enhances erectile function. Conversely, strength training activities enhance general fitness and may have a secondary benefit for sexual health. Exercise regimens that combine both cardiovascular and muscle-strengthening activities should be balanced for those who want to use exercise as a means of treating ED. Including physical activity in one's routine helps with psychological well-being by lowering stress and anxiety, which are frequently associated with eating disorders. It also treats the physical aspects of eating disorders.

The complex relationship that exists between stress, sleep, and sexual health is an additional aspect of lifestyle adjustments related to treating eating disorders. Lack of sleep has been linked to hormonal abnormalities, such as a drop-in testosterone levels, which can exacerbate ED. Therefore, getting enough sleep is essential to treating erectile dysfunction holistically. It has long been known that stress—both psychological and physical—plays a major role in the development of ED. Stress management strategies, such mindfulness meditation and relaxation exercises, have demonstrated potential in easing the symptoms of ED by lessening the negative effects of stressors on the physiological functions of the body. The correlation shown between stress management and sleep quality highlights the need of adopting a holistic lifestyle approach in the treatment of ED.

dietary changes, consistent exercise, and efficient stress and sleep management are all important lifestyle choices that are essential to conquering erectile dysfunction.

Taking a comprehensive approach to treating ED that takes into account its psychological and physiological components improves overall health and offers a long-term framework for controlling and preventing this common illness.

CHAPTER SIX
PSYCHOLOGICAL METHODS
Therapy & Counseling

When it comes to treating and recovering from erectile dysfunction (ED), counseling and therapy are essential. This method acknowledges the relationship between psychological and physiological elements that affect sexual wellness. In counseling, individuals or couples examine the relational and emotional factors that lead to ED in collaboration with qualified professionals. To explore underlying problems, therapists frequently use interpersonal, psychodynamic, or psychoanalytic techniques. Therapists assist people in expressing worries and anxieties about their sexuality by encouraging open communication, which creates a secure environment for introspection and understanding. In order to lessen psychological obstacles impeding sexual function and performance anxiety, interpersonal dynamics and emotional intimacy are being explored. Additionally, counseling offers a forum for talking about lifestyle choices that can aggravate ED, like substance abuse or stress. A complete treatment approach that include therapy addresses the entire aspect of sexual health and promotes long-term healing.

CBT, Or Cognitive-Behavioral Therapy

One of the most popular psychological interventions for people with erectile dysfunction is cognitive-behavioral therapy (CBT). The goal of this method is to recognize and change the harmful mental patterns and actions that underlie sexual issues. CBT promotes a more positive outlook that is beneficial to sexual well-being by assisting people in identifying and challenging false ideas about performance, body image, and sexuality. Through planned sessions, therapists assist clients in creating coping mechanisms for the stress and anxiety that are frequently linked to eating disorders.

In order to promote a positive feedback loop of increased confidence and sexual function, cognitive behavioral therapy (CBT) aims to interrupt the cycle of negative beliefs that cause anxiety related to sexual performance.

Sensate concentration exercises are another component of CBT that can help people re-establish a connection with their bodies and encourage calm in intimate situations. Through the treatment of cognitive and behavioral components, CBT enables people to take charge of their ED, improving their overall confidence and level of sexual satisfaction.

Techniques For Relaxation And Mindfulness

The integration of mindfulness and relaxation techniques provides a comprehensive strategy for resolving erectile dysfunction by addressing the mind-body connection. Based on meditation techniques, mindfulness enables people to develop judgment-free present-moment awareness. People can reduce anxiety and performance pressure during sexual encounters by practicing mindfulness, which promotes a more open and relaxed mood. To encourage general relaxation and lower stress, mindfulness-based therapy frequently include methods like progressive muscle relaxation, guided imagery, and deep breathing. These behaviors directly affect the physiological reactions connected to sexual function in addition to improving psychological health. The best physiological conditions for sexual arousal and function are produced by mindfulness and relaxation practices, which decrease sympathetic nervous system activation and increase parasympathetic activity. By incorporating these techniques into daily life, one can improve general stress management, which will have a beneficial impact on one's sexual health and help one overcome erectile dysfunction.

psychological strategies for overcoming erectile dysfunction include cognitive-behavioral therapy, mindfulness, and relaxation methods.

The complex interactions between psychological and physiological elements that lead to ED are addressed by each of these therapies. Through open dialogue and the investigation of emotional and relational dynamics, counseling fosters understanding and lessens performance anxiety. The goals of cognitive-behavioral therapy are to break the loop of worry connected to performance, improve confidence, and recognize and change harmful thought patterns and behaviors. Through the promotion of present-moment awareness and the creation of an ideal physiological environment for sexual function, mindfulness and relaxation techniques offer a comprehensive approach. By incorporating these psychological techniques into an all-encompassing treatment program, people can take on the complex nature of erectile dysfunction and work toward long-term improvements in their sexual health and well-being.

CHAPTER SEVEN
SUGGESTIONS AND ALTERNATIVE THERAPIES

A common ailment that affects men all over the world, erectile dysfunction (ED) may be extremely distressing and negatively influence a person's general quality of life. Although the mainstay of ED treatment has been pharmaceutical interventions such as phosphodiesterase type 5 (PDE5) inhibitors, interest in complementary and alternative therapies is expanding. Three different approaches are examined in this section: acupuncture, yoga, and meditation, as well as herbal supplements.

Supplements With Herbs

For decades, many traditional medical systems have used herbal supplements to treat sexual health issues, including ED.

Some plants are thought to have aphrodisiac qualities and may be good for erectile dysfunction.

For example, ginseng has been researched for its vasodilatory properties and effects on nitric oxide synthesis, which is important for penile blood flow. It has been proposed that horny goat weed, another plant, has PDE5 inhibitory effects that are comparable to those of prescription drugs.

It is important to recognize the scant scientific data and possible hazards linked with herbal supplements, even in cases where research yield encouraging findings. Thorough research, quality control, and dosage standardization are crucial for proving the effectiveness and safety of these treatments.

The Use Of Acupuncture

A crucial part of traditional Chinese medicine, acupuncture stimulates qi flow by inserting tiny needles into predetermined body locations. Acupuncture for ED seeks to promote general health, treat underlying imbalances, and improve sexual function. Numerous investigations have looked into the possible advantages of acupuncture in treating ED, and the findings point to better erectile function and satisfaction. Although the exact processes underlying these effects are unknown, it has been suggested that acupuncture may have an impact on hormonal balance, neurovascular pathways, and psychological aspects. To determine acupuncture's involvement in treating ED, including the best treatment plans and long-term results, additional excellent research is necessary.

Meditation And Yoga

Sexual health is greatly influenced by the mind-body link, and therapies such as yoga and meditation aim to achieve balance between the mental and physical spheres of health. Yoga has been investigated as a possible treatment option for ED because of its emphasis on conscious breathing, particular postures, and controlled breathing. According to certain research, yoga can help erectile dysfunction by increasing blood flow, lowering stress levels, and encouraging relaxation. In a similar vein, meditation's capacity to reduce stress may have a favorable influence on sexual health. Mindfulness-based therapies have demonstrated potential in reducing psychological issues including anxiety and stress associated to performance that contribute to eating disorders. Although these methods provide a comprehensive viewpoint, further thorough research is required to determine their efficacy, pinpoint best practices, and comprehend the mechanisms by which they affect sexual function.

In conclusion, a multifaceted approach to treating this complicated problem is reflected in the investigation of herbal cures and alternative therapies for erectile dysfunction. Acupuncture, yoga, meditation, and herbal supplements all present different viewpoints and possible advantages. But it's crucial to approach these medicines critically, acknowledging the gaps in the available scientific data and the need for more investigation. To guarantee the greatest outcomes for patients struggling with this difficult disease, integrating these alternative techniques into conventional ED management necessitates thorough evaluation, standardization, and coordination between traditional and modern medical practices.

CHAPTER EIGHT
CHANGES IN LIFESTYLE FOR LONG-TERM HEALTH

The common disorder known as erectile dysfunction (ED) can have a serious negative effect on a person's quality of life. A complete approach is needed to treat ED, and changing one's lifestyle is essential to controlling the illness and promoting long-term health. Three key areas of lifestyle change will be covered in this discussion: managing weight, cutting back on alcohol, and quitting smoking.

Quitting Smoking

One known risk factor for ED is smoking. Smoking's negative impact on vascular health is a major factor in how it affects erectile performance. Tobacco products contain nicotine, which narrows blood vessels and lowers blood flow to all parts of the body, including the vaginal area.

Additionally, smoking worsens blood flow by promoting the growth of atherosclerosis, a disorder marked by the accumulation of fatty deposits in arteries. Another side effect of smoking is endothelial dysfunction, which damages the lining of blood arteries and prevents them from dilatation, which further impedes proper blood flow. As a result, using smoking cessation techniques is essential to reducing these negative consequences and enhancing erectile performance.

Moderation In Alcohol Consumption

While moderate alcohol use is usually regarded as appropriate, excessive consumption can have detrimental effects on sexual health and may even cause ED to develop or worsen. Because alcohol depresses the central nervous system, it may make it more difficult for the brain to communicate signs of sexual arousal. Chronic alcohol misuse can also result in hormone imbalances that impact testosterone levels and, in turn, erectile function. Additionally, alcohol is linked to the development of liver cirrhosis, which can have a negative effect on sexual health and cause hormonal abnormalities. In order to prevent or treat ED, one must lead a moderately alcohol-consuming lifestyle that promotes balance and protects one's sexual and physical health.

Control Of Weight

An established risk factor for ED, obesity has a variety of effects on sexual health. Overweight is a factor in the development of metabolic syndrome, which is a group of disorders that includes insulin resistance, dyslipidemia, and high blood pressure. These disorders are all linked to the pathophysiology of ED. Moreover, oxidative stress and inflammation linked to obesity might negatively impact blood vessel function and jeopardize erectile function. Distress related to body image and low self-esteem are among the psychological effects of obesity that can exacerbate sexual dysfunction.

Thus, adopting weight-management techniques, such as a healthy diet and frequent exercise, is essential to treating the underlying causes of eating disorders and advancing general health.

To sum up, modifying one's lifestyle is essential to treating erectile dysfunction holistically. Restoring and maintaining sexual health is facilitated by quitting smoking, consuming alcohol in moderation, and controlling one's weight.

By putting these lifestyle changes into practice, you not only treat the immediate causes of ED but also lay the groundwork for long-term wellbeing.

Those who struggle with ED should view these lifestyle adjustments as foundational elements for building a healthier, more satisfying life, rather than just as therapies.

CHAPTER NINE
NAVIGATING RELATIONSHIPS
Honest Communication

In order to treat and overcome erectile dysfunction (ED) in a relationship, open communication is essential. It is critical that partners have open and sympathetic discussions about the difficulties they are having when it comes to ED. This entails having judgment-free conversations about worries, anxieties, and feelings associated with ED.

A supportive environment where both parties feel heard and understood is created via clear communication. It is crucial to create an environment where talking about sexual health is accepted, as this will enable more candid conversations regarding the origins and potential fixes of problems. Encouraging openness fosters a cooperative effort to resolve the problem by easing tension and fear about ED.

Beyond Sexual Intimacy

Even though physical closeness plays a significant role in romantic relationships, it's just as crucial to acknowledge and foster other forms of connection. In the process of overcoming erectile dysfunction, partners can investigate and improve their emotional and psychological bonds.

This entails doing things like having meaningful conversations, taking up hobbies together, and spending quality time together that promote a stronger emotional connection.

Couples can find other means of expressing their love and affection by moving the emphasis away from performance-oriented expectations. Increasing emotional closeness can make a relationship more robust and enjoyable in general, as well as lessen the strain that comes with sexual performance.

Relationship Guidance

One useful tool for negotiating the difficulties of erectile dysfunction in a relationship is relationship counseling.

Getting professional advice from a sexual health-trained therapist or counselor can provide a regulated and encouraging setting for couples to discuss their issues. Couples can discuss the psychological and interpersonal aspects of ED in a therapeutic context. To meet the unique requirements of the couple, counselors can offer behavioral interventions, communication techniques, and coping strategies. In addition to providing a forum for addressing any underlying problems that might be aggravating the effects of ED on the partnership, relationship counseling also fosters a cooperative attitude to overcoming obstacles and advances the general well-being of the relationship.

CHAPTER TEN
UPCOMING ADVANCEMENTS AND STUDIES

Men's health has long been concerned with erectile dysfunction (ED), and current research is working to identify novel treatments and provide insight into the underlying causes of this problem. For those who are dealing with ED, there is hope thanks to newly developed medicines. One of these is the investigation of gene therapy, a novel field with promise for addressing the genetic reasons of erectile dysfunction. Researchers hope to create long-lasting medicines with fewer side effects than traditional methods by focusing on particular genes linked to vascular health and erectile function.

Further efforts are being made to introduce new compounds and improve the efficacy of currently available drugs through pharmacological improvements.

PDE5 inhibitors, such tadalafil and sildenafil, have completely changed the way that ED is treated. However, research is still being done to increase the effectiveness of these medications and create alternatives that have fewer negative effects. In addition, research into stem cell therapy and other forms of regenerative medicine is gaining momentum as a possible treatment option for damaged tissue and the restoration of normal erectile function. There is hope for a more all-encompassing and long-lasting approach to ED management in this field of study.

Current Erectile Dysfunction Research

Numerous current studies are being conducted in the dynamic and ever-evolving field of erectile dysfunction research in an effort to better understand the complex nature of this disorder. Relationship between ED and cardiovascular health is one important topic of focus. Scholars are investigating the complex relationships that exist between endothelial dysfunction, which is a risk factor for cardiovascular disease, and its effects on erectile dysfunction. Knowing these links can help with preventative strategies and integrated methods to treating heart problems and ED.

Additionally, researchers are looking into the involvement of the central and peripheral nerve systems in erectile function as they examine the neurogenic factors impacting ED. This entails researching the intricate interactions that neurotransmitters, hormones, and brain circuits have in order to provide insights into possible targets for therapy. Furthermore, research is being done on psychological factors that contribute to ED, recognizing the reciprocal relationship between mental health and erectile function.

The goal of this field of research is to create treatments that deal with the psychological components of ED, offering a more all-encompassing method of care.

CONCLUSION

The field of erectile dysfunction is changing as a result of important advancements in science and the introduction of cutting-edge therapeutic approaches. The investigation of gene therapy, advances in pharmaceuticals, and regenerative medicine point to a paradigm shift in the strategy for treating ED from the ground up.

For those dealing with this common and frequently stigmatized ailment, these novel treatments offer hope for a more tailored and successful management of erectile dysfunction.

The intricacy of erectile dysfunction and the need for a comprehensive understanding are highlighted by the continuous study in this field. Understanding the relationships among neurogenic variables, cardiovascular health, and psychosocial influences on erectile function is important for developing a comprehensive understanding of ED. This information not only helps to improve current treatment approaches, but it also opens the door for novel interventions that take into account the interdependence of the neurological, psychological, and physical facets of sexual health.

As we move to the future, bringing these improvements from the lab to clinical practice will require cooperation between researchers, medical practitioners, and pharmaceutical innovators.

It is critical to close the gap between scientific advancement and readily available, patient-focused erectile dysfunction treatments.

By doing this, the medical community will be able to offer people less intrusive, more individualized, and more successful choices for controlling ED, which will eventually improve the quality of life for those who suffer from this common ailment.